THE HYPERTENSION COOKBOOK FOR BEGINNERS

500 Recipes for Quick and Easy Low-Carb Homemade Cooking

Dr. Julia S. Gerald

Table of Contents

Introduction

High blood pressure is referred to as hypertension in medicine. Although the two phrases are sometimes used interchangeably, "high blood pressure" generally refers to a measurement that is persistently over 140/90 mmHg. When the systolic (top number) or diastolic (bottom number) readings are regularly between 120 and 139 or 80 and 89, respectively, the term "pre-hypertension" or "pre-hypertensive" is used. Pre-hypertensive people have a higher risk of developing high blood pressure.

Important Hypertension

Essential hypertension is the phrase used to describe excessive blood pressure when the underlying cause cannot be identified. Additionally, it is known as "primary hypertension." 90–95 percent of people with high blood pressure have been identified as having essential hypertension. A sickness with no apparent etiology is sometimes referred to as "idiopathic" in medicine.

Subsequent Hypertension

Secondary hypertension is the diagnosis when the exact etiology of hypertension is known or established. This diagnosis may be the outcome of many medical conditions, such as:

- Side effects of medication
- Various malignancies and tumors
- Kidney issues
- Pregnancy
- Gestational hypertension

During pregnancy, hypertension is a frequent medical condition. The four subtypes of this kind of hypertension are as follows:

Preeclampsia-eclampsia

The presence of persistent hypertension and preeclampsia.

The more precise description is now known as "gestational hypertension," which has replaced the previous phrase "pregnancy-induced hypertension."

Preeclampsia and toxemia, diseases of gestational hypertension, cause more than 500,000 newborn fatalities and 76,000 maternal deaths each year.

Hypertension in United States

In the United States, hypertension claimed the lives of almost 56,000 individuals in 2006. Adults with hypertension make up one in three (about 74.5 million people).

In 2006, 77.6% of people with hypertension were aware of their disease; yet, only 67.9% were receiving treatment, more than 44% had it under control, and more than 55% didn't. Between 1996 and 2006, the number of fatalities from hypertension climbed by 48.1%, while the mortality rate increased by 19.5%.

Compared to those using calcium channel blockers, patients taking a specific beta-blocker had a 51% higher risk of developing newly diagnosed diabetes. When using high blood pressure drugs, be sure to carefully evaluate the many unfavorable side effects. When treating one ailment, a drug will often have lethal or severe negative effects on another.

Statistics on Adverse Drug Reactions (ADRs)

- Each year, there are more than 2 million significant ADRs.

- ADRs result in more than 106,000 fatalities per year.

- Patients living in nursing homes experience 350,000 ADRs.

It is dangerous to combine prescription and over-the-counter (OTC) medications. When combined with a narcotic substance, OTC medications that include alcohol and antihistamine reduce the heart rate and stifle respiration, rendering them fatal.

Eliminating the causes should be your primary focus if you have hypertension. Everyone else's main priority should be prevention. Learning how one little toxin, which is present in a variety of consumables, might impact your blood pressure and health, is the first step. You can regulate your blood pressure and your health by eliminating it from your life.

Part One: Hypertension 101

What You Need to Know

High blood pressure (HBP), usually referred to as hypertension, is a significant medical disease. It occurs when your blood's rushing through your arteries with an excessive amount of power. Blood is pushed through your arteries to the rest of your body as your heart beats. Your blood pressure increases when the blood presses harder against the artery walls. Your blood pressure may vary during the day. It is often greater in the morning, after exercise, or during stressful times.

It's common to have increased blood pressure for brief periods. However, if your blood pressure is consistently high, it might lead to major health issues. By using a monitor at home and talking to your doctor, you can keep tabs on your blood pressure. An adult's typical resting reading is at 120/80 mm HG.

If HBP is not managed or identified, it may be fatal. It may result in peripheral artery disease, angina, heart failure, stroke, heart attack, kidney disease or failure, vision loss, sexual dysfunction, or kidney failure. These illnesses need to be addressed since they are so dangerous. When to call your doctor may be determined by being aware of the symptoms and indicators.

What are the most prevalent symptoms and indicators of hypertension?

- The back of your head is giving you a severe headache.
- Abnormally low strength.
- Anxiety may manifest as both mental and bodily restlessness.
- Accompanying tension or anxiety and dizziness
- Buzzing or ringing in the persistent ears.

Because of the involvement of the brain, a lack of sleep is known as insomnia.

Tiny blood vessels in the nose might burst as a result of increased pressure, causing nosebleeds. Sensation as if your breathing is about to stop due to shortness of breath.

Physical effort may cause chest pains, particularly along the left chest wall, in the shoulder or neck area, when the heart muscles are deprived of blood and oxygen.

Fainting or a sensation that things are moving all around you. Alterations in the capillary blood capillaries in the eyes that affect vision.

Why does hypertension occur?

- Family background
- Obesity
- Excessive booze consumption
- Sedentary behavior/lack of activity
- A diet heavy in fat or salt
- and high caffeine consumption
- Stress and smoking.

How is hypertension managed?

- Reduce your weight and keep an eye on your waistline. One of the best methods for treating hypertension outside medicine is weight loss. Additionally, having a large waistline might raise your risk for hypertension. To find out what a healthy waist measurement is, see your doctor.

- Frequent exercise—If you have pre-hypertension, regular exercise for at least 30 minutes a day may help decrease your blood pressure or keep it from rising. Some of the finest workouts for decreasing blood pressure are walking, running, swimming, cycling, and weight training. Consult your doctor before beginning an exercise program.

- Eat well-balanced meals that are high in fruits, vegetables, whole grains, and low-fat dairy products to help decrease your blood pressure. Reduce your caffeine intake.

- Reduce salt intake; even a slight reduction in salt consumption may result in a 2–8 mm Hg drop in blood pressure. Some folks should cut down on salt even more since they are more sensitive to it. All African Americans over the age of 51, those with high blood pressure, diabetes, or chronic renal disease fall under this category.

- Reduce alcohol consumption, and stop smoking. You may lower your blood pressure by giving up smoking.

- Reduce Stress: HBP may be exacerbated by long-term stress. If you often resort to bad eating choices, drinking, or even smoking, occasional stress might also be a concern.

- Making regular doctor visits may aid in the monitoring and treatment of HBP. If none of the previous choices work to bring your blood pressure down to a healthy level, a prescription drug may be given to you.

It's important to get medical attention for hypertension since it may be dangerous. Regular blood pressure checks and paying attention to your body's signals may save your life. Pay close attention to the symptoms and indications of hypertension, and get in touch with your doctor if any appear.

High Blood Pressure and Pregnant Women

Pregnancy-related high blood pressure is a dangerous condition that puts both your life and the life of your unborn child at peril. Nearly 15% of all pregnancies in the US are affected by the illness, often known as maternal hypertension. Hospitalization is necessary for several pregnancy-related high blood pressure complications:

Eclampsia: Pregnancy-related high blood pressure seizures Strokes: Interruption of blood supply to the brain, resulting in weakness and irreversible incapacity Preeclampsia: Pregnancy-related high blood pressure that puts stress on the heart and other organs such the liver, kidneys, lungs, and eyes

Premature delivery: the need for the baby to be delivered early than anticipated before growth and development are finished in the womb. Placental abruption: The separation of the baby's blood supply (placenta) from the uterine wall

High Blood Pressure and the Risk of Pregnancy-Related Death

Even if you've never had high blood pressure before, it may occur during pregnancy. Gestational hypertension is the medical term for the situation. Chronic hypertension is high blood pressure that you already have before being pregnant. You run a higher chance of having harmful consequences both during and just after pregnancy if you have either form of high blood pressure.

According to research conducted by the Centers for Disease Control and Prevention in 2022, roughly one-third of Americans who died during delivery between 2017 and 2019 had excessive blood pressure. The majority of them had become ill while pregnant.

According to Rutgers research, the risk of dying from a high blood pressure-related consequence is higher if you are over 45 and/or medically obese. Additionally, Black individuals are at a heightened risk of dying during pregnancy from a high blood pressure-related reason because they are more likely to have high blood pressure-related health issues as a result of systemic racism. Therefore, knowing how to lower your risk of high blood pressure-related issues before, during, and after pregnancy is crucial – particularly if you currently have high blood pressure or are at a high risk of developing it.

Before Conception

Do all in your power to maintain a healthy body weight and keep active if you already have a history of high blood pressure. Discuss with your healthcare practitioner how to manage your high blood pressure as well as the safety of your medicines during pregnancy.

Take steps to lower your stress level and look after your mental health. Stress and worry have been connected to gestational hypertension and may raise blood pressure.

The lack of sleep and sleep apnea may both contribute to hypertension. Therefore, if you don't feel refreshed in the mornings or aren't getting enough sleep, speak to your doctor about what you can do to enhance your sleep.

Additionally, if you have had preeclampsia during pregnancy, you are more likely to experience it in subsequent pregnancies. Please talk to your physician about your specific preeclampsia risk.

When you are expecting

Make sure your provider is aware of your high blood pressure if you get pregnant. Attend all of your planned checks, as they advised.

Using a home monitor, you may also periodically check your blood pressure on your own. It's far preferable to find out sooner rather than later if it begins to rise over your usual blood pressure level. You may get support from your provider to maintain control. Consult your insurer to see whether your health insurance will at least partly cover a blood pressure monitor.

Continue to consume wholesome meals and keep an eye on your weight. Your chance of acquiring hypertension or seeing it worsen may be decreased as a result.

Preeclampsia

Preeclampsia symptoms to be on the lookout for include: nausea and vomiting; headaches; eye issues like light sensitivity or black spots in your eyesight; belly discomfort; swelling in your hands and face; shortness of breath; and a general sensation of being sick.

Some of these signs and symptoms, such as nausea and vomiting, may occur throughout normal pregnancy. However, it's best to see a doctor right once if you see a dramatic shift.

Abrupt Placentation

Third-trimester pregnancy is when placental abruption is most likely to occur. This critical problem might endanger your life or the life of your unborn child.

Vaginal bleeding, back and/or belly pain, discomfort or stiffness in the womb, contractions that are often close together, and a decrease in the baby's activity are all possible symptoms.

If you have any of these signs, consult a doctor straight soon to determine if you need hospitalization. If an early birth is required, your doctor may prescribe medication to regulate your blood pressure as well as another medication to aid in the development of your baby's lungs.

You will require an emergency delivery, most likely by cesarean section, if the abruption is severe or poses a health risk to you or your unborn child (C-section). In case of an emergency, dial 911 right away.

Following Delivery

After your baby is delivered, preeclampsia may still occur, often within the first 48 hours but sometimes even up to six weeks or later. So, if you have any symptoms, let your doctor know right away. You could need urgent medical attention.

When blood pressure is not under control before, during, or after pregnancy, a stroke may occur. Strokes are still possible twelve or more weeks after birth, even if the high blood pressure was caused during the pregnancy. Keep an eye out for abrupt

• Vision issues, numbness in your face, arm, or leg, particularly on one side of your body; confusion, difficulty speaking or understanding people;

• Loss of coordination or balance

• A severe headache with no apparent reason

Call 911 right away if you suspect you're suffering a stroke so that an ambulance can take you to the hospital emergency department. Minutes matter!

If you have pregnant hypertension, you run the risk of developing persistent hypertension after giving birth. You should treat this with the help of your primary care physician since it may increase your lifelong risk of developing heart, brain, eye, and kidney illnesses. Future high-risk pregnancies may potentially result from it.

Also, remember to take care of your emotional well-being. High blood pressure during pregnancy increases the likelihood of postpartum depression, anxiety, and post-traumatic stress disorder. Furthermore, you and your newborn kid may become at grave risk as a result of these mental health issues.

Obstetric difficulties might result from high blood pressure. However, keeping both you and your unborn child healthy may be achieved by working with your doctor to monitor and regulate your blood pressure and being aware of the warning signals to look out for.

Adapting to the New Life

High blood pressure, often known as hypertension, is a dangerous medical disease that is prevalent among Americans. Despite being a significant medical disease, hypertension may be managed. The greatest thing is that you may not even need medication to lower your blood pressure.

High-Risk Categories & High Blood Pressure

Everyone has hypertension, but there are a few factors that will put you in considerable danger. Smoking, eating poorly, being overweight, and not exercising all raise risk. Changing a few aspects of your lifestyle may help you manage your blood pressure if you have been diagnosed with hypertension. You might ask the doctor at the health center in east Texas whether it's feasible to lower your blood pressure naturally. It is in numerous instances.

Beginning an exercise regimen

With hypertension, beginning an exercise program need a little more caution. Although you want to avoid overstressing your body, you also want to slightly exceed your physical limitations. In your first session, don't attempt to take on too much, but you must push yourself beyond your comfort zone. A heart rate monitor could be a smart purchase, depending on your physical condition. Discuss the safe heart rate range with your doctor and exercise within it. Increase your workout routine as you get more comfortable with it. Exercise is a fantastic technique to start lowering your blood pressure.

Making Dietary Changes

There is a very strong likelihood that your food has contributed to your "hypertension" if you experience it. Controlling your weight and blood pressure is a lot easier when healthy food and exercise are combined. Preservatives and high-sodium foods should be avoided. Put the salt shaker away, don't slather on the salad dressing, and steer clear of meals heavy in saturated fats. You don't have to stop eating your favorite foods, but you do need to regulate them. Avoid rewarding yourself with junk food as a reward for eating well. You'll find it simpler to stick with healthy eating if you make a long-term commitment to it.

Quit smoking.

Everyone is aware at this point that smoking is harmful to one's health. The harm cigarettes do to the body is subtle. The best ways to stop smoking have been advocated by several groups. Some individuals discover that they need nicotine patches, but others find that quitting "cold turkey"—completely—and overcoming the withdrawal symptoms on their own—has the greatest results. Nicotine patches are effective if you find going cold turkey too challenging.

Mastering Your Health

Most of us will eventually develop high blood pressure, sometimes known as hypertension. This is a frequent condition that, if the proper measures are not taken to treat and prevent it, may worsen with time. Although a lot of people believe that having high blood pressure might cause mortality, this isn't always the case. You may still have a regular life, but you must act differently. This article breaks out how to manage hypertension and maintain a healthy, happy lifestyle.

Study Hypertension.

High blood pressure is often seen as an old-age condition. But in reality, it may have an impact on people of any age. The greatest treatment when it comes to your health is prevention. It will be more difficult to lower your blood pressure the longer you wait to get therapy.

Heart disease and stroke risk factors include high blood pressure. It is also a dangerous disorder that, if ignored, may result in renal failure, blindness, and other problems.

With approximately 50 million Americans reported to have high blood pressure, the number of individuals afflicted by hypertension is increasing. Many of them are unaware of it.

Kate Carnell, CEO of the Heart Foundation, claims that many individuals with high blood pressure are ignorant about the risks involved with the disease and the harm it may do over time. In a statement, she said that "we need to increase awareness about this ailment and its related symptoms among community members." People must be aware of the steps they may take to lower the danger.

People with high blood pressure may benefit from a variety of therapies, including medication and lifestyle modifications including losing weight, managing stress, and exercising. You can manage your hypertension while maintaining your health with a little effort.

Consult your physician.

When you have high blood pressure, the blood is pressurized in your blood vessels more than it should be. However, there are things you can do to manage your blood pressure and reduce your risk of heart disease and stroke.

Your heart has to work harder to pump blood through your body if you have high blood pressure. Your heart suffers harm as a result, and it functions less effectively. You have a higher risk of having a stroke or developing kidney disease if you have high blood pressure.

Together with your doctor, you may come up with a strategy that reduces your risk by changing your lifestyle and taking medicine. You may minimize your risk of heart disease and stroke, protect yourself from the risks of uncontrolled high blood pressure, and bring your blood pressure under control.

Follow your statistics

When you consistently experience systolic readings of 140 mm Hg or higher or diastolic readings of 90 mm Hg or above, your blood pressure is regarded as high. According to a study, if you have persistently high blood pressure readings of 130/80 mm Hg or greater as an adult or kid aged 13 or older, your doctor may also diagnose you with high blood pressure.

Your doctor will likely take a third measurement to confirm the diagnosis if your blood pressure has been over the normal range for up to two readings (taken at different appointments). You will be given a high blood pressure diagnosis if the average of these three values is more than 140/90 mm Hg.

It's crucial to obtain regular examinations since high blood pressure often has no symptoms.

Watch your diet

We all understand the benefits of eating a balanced diet for our bodies, but it's also crucial for controlling blood pressure. This is particularly true if you have hypertension or high blood pressure.

The DASH diet is an eating regimen designed to decrease or manage high blood pressure. The DASH diet encourages several meals that may decrease blood pressure. Fruits, vegetables, whole grains, and dairy products free or low in fat are a few of them. The DASH diet also restricts sugary meals and drinks as well as foods and beverages rich in saturated fats, such as fatty meats, full-fat dairy products, and tropical oils including coconut, palm kernel, and palm oils. You may decrease your blood pressure by around 5 points in only two weeks by following the DASH diet.

Researchers and medical professionals have discovered that certain meals may lower blood pressure. These include meals high in protein, fiber, potassium, and magnesium.

The following meals are some of the best for lowering blood pressure:

- Avocados: This pears-shaped fruit's flesh is a good source of monounsaturated fats, which may decrease cholesterol levels. Avocados contain almost twice as much potassium per ounce as bananas.

- Yogurt and low-fat or fat-free milk: The calcium and vitamin D in these dairy products help maintain healthy bones and may lower the risk of osteoporosis. Additionally, the protein in fat-free or low-fat milk may help you feel fuller for longer.

- Lentils and beans: In every meal, beans and lentils are a fantastic source of protein and a tasty alternative to meat. Additionally, they contain a lot of fiber, which might prolong your feeling of fullness. Additionally, they include magnesium and potassium, which might help decrease blood pressure.

Exercise.

People with high blood pressure often use drugs to reduce their pressure. But exercise is also a vital component of life. You may lower your high blood pressure and lose extra weight with its assistance.

The American Heart Association (AHA) advises engaging in at least 30 minutes of moderate-intensity aerobic exercise for a total of 150 minutes, at least five days a week. Exercises at this level range from brisk walking to swimming and lawn mowing. Running and aerobic dance are examples of vigorous-intensity aerobic exercise. The American Heart Association advises 75 minutes of aerobic exercise, spread out over three days, comprising at least 25 minutes of strenuous activity, or a mix of moderate and vigorous activity.

The AHA advises doing strengthening activities at least twice a week in addition to aerobic exercise. Examples include employing resistance bands and lifting free weights.

Before beginning an exercise regimen, see your doctor if you haven't been active lately. Activities that are suitable for your health and degree of fitness might be suggested by your doctor.

Consume alcohol in moderation.

If you have hypertension, you may want to cut down on your alcohol intake.

Going cold turkey is not a smart idea, however. Cutting down too rapidly on alcohol if you're accustomed to it might cause withdrawal symptoms like sleeplessness and trembling hands.

For ladies, start with one drink and for males, start with two. Drink nonalcoholic drinks in between alcoholic ones to stay within your daily limit.

Remember that 5 ounces of wine are comparable to 12 ounces of beer or 1.5 ounces of 80-proof distilled spirits if you decide to drink wine (such as vodka, cognac, or rum).

Drinking too much raises your chance of acquiring the illness even if your blood pressure is not elevated.

Additionally, it increases your chance of developing some malignancies, heart failure, liver cirrhosis, and other health issues.

Be less stressed

It's crucial to lessen stress in your life if you have high blood pressure. A heart attack or stroke may result from persistent stress. Your arteries may constrict over time as a result of the stress hormone cortisol, which raises your chance of developing high blood pressure.

There are several approaches to stress reduction. Consider the following, for instance:

- Enjoy yourself and life more. Visit relatives and pets, go out with friends, watch comedic movies, and read literature that makes you chuckle. Your blood pressure may be lowered by laughter.
- Sleep for seven to eight hours every night. If you're having trouble sleeping, discuss solutions with your doctor.

- You could learn how to react more when you're stressed out by using relaxation methods. This has the same effect on blood pressure reduction as prescription medicines. Meditation, deep breathing exercises, and guided visualization are all examples of relaxation methods.

Giving up smoking

One of the most important things you can do to enhance your health and reduce your risk of heart disease is to stop smoking.

The advantages of quitting smoking begin right away. Your pulse rate and blood pressure have already started to decrease after just 20 minutes.

In fact, during the first year after quitting permanently, your risk for a heart attack lowers significantly. The advantages keep expanding in the long run. Your life expectancy may increase by up to years and your risk of having a stroke decrease.

It's never too late to stop using tobacco. Even if you've been a smoker for a long time, giving up may improve your health. Even if you're already feeling the effects of smoking, your body will start healing itself straight immediately.

Organize a network of loved ones and friends for support.

You are not alone yourself. You may control your hypertension and achieve your objectives for a healthy lifestyle with the support of lifestyle modifications, medicines, and stress management.

If you're having trouble controlling your hypertension, your family and friends can help you emotionally. According to research, those with great social support from their families, friends, or religious organizations often have a lower blood pressure than those who do not.

Having a solid support system is one of the most crucial aspects of controlling your high blood pressure. Both individuals who can assist you with physical duties and those who will provide emotional support are included in this.

What to look for in a system of assistance

It's useful to turn to friends and family who can support you while you're attempting to control hypertension and make big lifestyle adjustments. These folks should ideally:

• be supportive of your objectives;

• be honest and upfront with you;

• be eager to learn about your condition and what is required to manage it;

• be able to help you out when you need it.

You shouldn't be prevented from leading a normal life by hypertension.

You may still lead a regular life with hypertension, but you will need to alter your lifestyle to be healthy.

Even if you feel well, you must take your medication every day, and you must also get your blood pressure tested often.

You must also be careful about how much salt you consume as well as what you eat and drink. You will also need to exercise more.

Your blood pressure may be controlled for the rest of your life with medication and a healthy lifestyle.

Part Two: 500 Recipes for Homemade

Breakfast Recipes

These dishes make it simple to have a nutritious, delicious breakfast even on hectic mornings. Bananas, dark leafy greens, and nuts are all excellent sources of potassium, magnesium, or calcium that may help decrease blood pressure.

Additionally, you won't have to spend the whole morning in the kitchen since dishes like our Smoked Salmon, Egg, & Pickled Beet Bagel Sandwich or Spinach & Egg Scramble with Raspberries can be prepared in 10 minutes or less.

Avocado-Spinach Smoothie

The frozen banana and avocado give this nutritious green smoothie a luxuriously creamy texture. Up to a day in advance, prepare it and keep it in the refrigerator until you need a vegetable boost.

Ingredients:

- 1 cup of nonfat plain yogurt;
- 2 tablespoons of water;
- 1 teaspoon of honey;
- 1 cup of fresh spinach;
- 1 frozen banana; and 1/4 avocado.

Directions:

In a blender, combine yogurt, spinach, banana, avocado, water, and honey. until smooth, puree.

Nutritional data:

Serving Size: 1 smoothie Each serving contains 357 calories, 17.7g of protein, 57.8g of carbohydrates, 7.8g of dietary fiber, 39.3g of sugar, 8.2g of fat, 1.5g of saturated fat, 4.9mg of cholesterol, 3832.7IU of vitamin A, 33.5mcg of vitamin C, 93.8mcg of folate, 554.1mg of calcium, 2.6mg of iron, 133.4mg of magnesium, 1294.8mg of

Exchanges: 1 1/2 nonfat milk, 1 1/2 fat, 1 1/2 fruit, 1/2 other carbohydrate, 1/2 vegetable

Breakfast with spinach and eggs with raspberries

One of the finest meals for weight reduction is this quick egg scramble with substantial toast. It mixes hearty whole-grain bread and spinach, which is rich in nutrients, with weight-loss superfoods eggs and raspberries. The total calorie count for the meal is slightly under 300, and the protein and fiber help you feel full.

Ingredients:

- 1 piece of whole-grain bread that has been toasted,
- 1 teaspoon of canola oil,
- 1 1/2 cups of baby spinach (1 1/2 ounces),
- 2 large eggs that have been softly beaten,
- a pinch of kosher salt, a pinch of ground pepper, and
- 1/2 cup of fresh raspberries.

Directions

- A small nonstick skillet with medium-high heat is used to heat the oil. Add the spinach and simmer for 1 to 2 minutes, stirring often, until wilted. Onto a platter, transfer the spinach.
- Clean the pan, then add eggs and cook it up over medium-low. Cook for 1 to 2 minutes, stirring once or twice to achieve uniform cooking. Add the spinach, salt, and pepper, and stir.
- Along with bread and strawberries, serve the scramble.

2 eggs, 1 piece of bread, and 1/2 cup of raspberries make up the serving.

Per serving, there are 296 calories, 17.8g of protein, 20.9g of carbohydrates, 7g of dietary fiber, 4.8g of sugars, 15.7g of fat, 3.7g of saturated fat, 372mg of cholesterol, 3312.6IU of vitamin A, 28.1mcg of vitamin

C, 79.4mcg of folate, 138.8mg of calcium, 4.2mg of iron, 76.1mg of magnesium, 292.6mg of potassium

Exchanges: 1 fat, 1/2 fruit, 1/2 starch, and 1/2 vegetable for the two medium-fat proteins.

Banana-Chocolate Protein Smoothie

This smoothie gets a dose of plant-based protein from red lentils. Use unsweetened coconut water or almond milk instead of the dairy milk in this smoothie to make it vegan.

Ingredients:

- A frozen banana;
- A half-cup of red lentils that have been cooked;
- A cup of nonfat milk; two teaspoons of unsweetened chocolate powder; and
- A teaspoon of pure maple syrup.

Directions:

Blend the banana, lentils, milk, chocolate, and syrup. until smooth, puree.

Nutritional data:

portion size Per serving of 1 smoothie, there are 310 calories, 15.3 grams of protein, 63.8 grams of carbohydrates, 8.5 grams of dietary fiber, 24.6 grams of sugar, 1.8 grams of fat, 0.6 grams of saturated fat, 2.5 milligrams of cholesterol, 347.7 IU of vitamin A, 10.9 milligrams of vitamin C, 109.2 milligrams of folate, 185.2 milligrams of calcium, 3.7 milligrams of iron, 87.3 milli

Exchanges: 1 lean protein, 1/2 nonfat milk, 1 starch, 2 fruits, and 1 other carbohydrate.

Banana-Blueberry Overnight Oats

The tastiest vegan overnight oats are made from regular oatmeal when it is combined with blueberries, a sweet banana, and creamy coconut milk. Prepare up to four jars at once and store them in the refrigerator for easy grab-and-go breakfasts all week.

Recipe:

Low-calorie, dairy-free, egg-free, gluten-free, vegetarian, vegan, nut-free, and soy-free nutrition profile

Ingredients:

- 12 cups unsweetened coconut milk,
- 12 cups old-fashioned oats (see tip),
- 12 tablespoons chia seeds (optional),
- 12 mashed bananas,
- 1 teaspoon maple syrup, 12 teaspoon salt,
- 12 cups fresh blueberries,
- 1 tablespoon unsweetened flakes coconut (Optional)

Directions:

In a pint-sized container, whisk together the coconut milk, oats, banana, maple syrup, salt, and chia seeds (if using). If desired, add blueberries and coconut to the top. Overnight, cover and chill.

Nutritional data:

1 1/2 cups per serving are the serving size. 285 calories, 6.2g of protein, 56.7g of carbs, 7.3g of dietary fiber, 19.6g of sugars, 5.7g of fat, 2.6g of saturated fat, 327.7IU of vitamin A, 12.3mcg of vitamin C, 47.7mcg of folate, 84.3mg of calcium, 1.8mg of iron, 81.8mg of magnesium, 452.4mg of potassium, 147.5mg of sodium, 0.2mg of

Replacements: 2 starch, 1 1/2 fruit, and 1/2 fat

Avocado with White Bean Toast

White beans and mashed avocado combine to create a creamy, fiber-rich topping that goes well with a crisp piece of bread. For a quick breakfast or snack, give it a

- **Ingredients:**
- 1 piece of whole-wheat bread, toasted;
- 1/4 avocado, mashed;

- 1/2 cup washed and drained canned white beans;
- Kosher salt to taste;
- Pinch each of ground pepper and salt;
- Pulverized red pepper

Directions:

White beans and mashed avocado go well on toast. Add a sprinkle of salt, pepper, and crushed red pepper to taste.

Nutritional data:

One slice per serving, please.

230 calories, 11.5g of protein, 34.7g of carbs, 11.3g of dietary fiber, 3g of sugar, 8.8g of fat, 1.3g of saturated fat, 74.2IU of vitamin A, 5.1mg of vitamin C, 158.2mcg of folate, 93.4mg of calcium, 2.3mg of iron, 35.1mg of magnesium, 655.4mg of potassium, 458.6mg of sodium, 0.1mg of this

Exchanges: 1 1/2 fat, 1 lean protein, 2 starch.

Egg and spinach tacos

For a quick, tasty breakfast, hard-boiled eggs are paired with spinach, cheese, and salsa. An avocado that has been mashed adds a creamy component, while a splash of lime juice adds acidity.

Ingredients:

- Two chopped hard-boiled eggs,
- two warmed corn tortillas, one cup chopped spinach,
- two tablespoons shredded Cheddar cheese,
- two tablespoons salsa,
- one-fourth of an avocado, one teaspoon lime juice,
- and a pinch of salt.

Directions

- In a small bowl, mash avocado and add salt and lime juice. Mix in the eggs.
- Place a portion of the mixture on each tortilla, then top with salsa, cheese, and 1/2 cup spinach.

Nutritional data

Serving Size: 2 tacos Each serving contains 421 calories, 21g of protein, 32g of carbs, 8g of dietary fiber, 3g of sugar, 24g of fat, 7g of saturated fat, 387mg of cholesterol, 658mg of sodium, and 564mg of potassium.

Banana and Kale Smoothie

This straightforward, pleasant, and adaptable kale and banana smoothie: Make a milkshake-like smoothie with cow's milk, add more sweetness with oat milk, or add more protein with nut milk.

Directions:

- Blend the kale, banana, honey, ice cubes, and milk (or non-dairy milk).
- Blend on medium-low speed, using the tamper if needed, until thoroughly incorporated.
- Increase speed to medium-high and blend until extremely smooth.

Nutritional data

266 calories, 5g of fat, 20mg of cholesterol, 129mg of sodium, 48g of carbs, 4g of dietary fiber, 10g of protein, 36g of sugars, 1mg of niacin equivalents, 3g of saturated fat, 2926IU of vitamin A, and 829mg of potassium.

Sandwich with smoked salmon, an egg, and pickled beets

Cucumbers, pickled beets, and fresh dill are added to this lox bagel riff in Scandinavian fashion for taste and texture.

Ingredients:

- 1 ounce of smoked salmon,
- sliced; 1/4 cup each of cucumber and pickled beets;
- 2 tablespoons cream cheese;
- 1 pumpernickel bagel thin or 2 slices pumpernickel bread, toasted;
- 1 big hard-boiled egg,
- sliced; and

- 1 tablespoon each of chopped fresh dill.

Directions

On 1 bagel, spread cream cheese and cut in half (or toast slice). Add salmon, cucumber, beets, and an egg as garnish. Top with the other thin half of the bagel and dill (or toast slice).

Nutritional data:

One sandwich per serving, serving size:

368 calories, 17g of fat, 222 mg of cholesterol, 631 mg of sodium, 35g of carbs, 2g of dietary fiber, 19g of protein, 11g of sugars, 3mg of niacin equivalents, 8g of saturated fat, 705 IU of vitamin A, and 334mg of potassium.

Migas with Spinach

In this variation of the Spanish meal Migas, spinach is added for color and nutrition, while sliced avocado adds a creamy texture.

Ingredients:

- Two big eggs,
- two cups of spinach,
- one chopped corn tortilla,
- one teaspoon of extra-virgin olive oil,
- two pinches of salt and pepper,
- two tablespoons of shredded Cheddar cheese, and
- one diced quarter of an avocado.

Directions

In a medium nonstick pan, heat the oil. Add the tortilla pieces and heat for three minutes, turning once, until crispy. For approximately a minute, while stirring, add the spinach and simmer until wilted. Add eggs to the pan after lightly beating them in a small dish with salt and pepper. About 2 minutes of stirring cooking will result in a set. Add the cheese, then turn off the heat. Add avocado on top.

Nutritional data:

One spinach Migas serving size equals:

402 calories, 21g of protein, 20g of carbs, 8g of dietary fiber, 1g of sugar, 27g of total fat, 8g of saturated fat, 386mg of cholesterol, 481mg of sodium, and 439mg of potassium.

Oats Overnight with Pumpkin

Use whatever nondairy milk you have on hand to make these simple vegan overnight oats. The recipe may be multiplied to provide nutritious breakfasts for the whole week. It's a terrific way to use up leftover canned pumpkins.

Ingredients:

Toasted pumpkin seeds or pecans are used as a garnish along with the following ingredients: 12 cups rolled oat,

13 cups unsweetened almond milk (or other non-dairy milk), 3 tablespoons pumpkin puree, 2 teaspoons pure maple syrup, 12 teaspoon vanilla extract, 14 teaspoon ground cinnamon, and a pinch of salt.

Directions

- In a pint-sized jar, combine the oats, milk, pumpkin, maple syrup, vanilla, cinnamon, and salt. Stir thoroughly. Overnight, cover and chill.
- If using, sprinkle pumpkin seeds (or nuts) over top before serving.

Nutritional data:

One jar's worth of food is one serving.

218 calories, 5.9g of protein, 40.8g of carbohydrates, 6g of dietary fiber, 10.9g of sugars, 4g of fat, 0.6g of saturated fat, 7316.2IU of vitamin A, 2mg of vitamin C, 25mcg of folate, 201mg of calcium, 2.3mg of iron,

54mg of magnesium, 290.4mg of potassium, 350.9mg of sodium, 0.2mg of thiamin, and 8g of

2 starches exchanged for 1 other carbohydrate

Tropical Greens Smoothie Packs with 3 Ingredients

Because frozen tropical fruit blends often include both mango and banana, which naturally add sweetness to smoothies, they provide an efficient shortcut. A fantastic approach to prevent fresh spinach from going bad before you can use it is to freeze it with fruit. Before mixing, feel free to add a scoop of your preferred protein powder.

Dietary Profile:

• Vegetarian Nutrition; Gluten-Free; Egg-Free; Nut-Free; Info

Ingredients

4 cups of fresh baby spinach, 1 (32-ounce) bag of frozen tropical fruit medley, and 4 cups of low-fat milk or a nondairy substitute divided.

Directions:

4 freezer-safe, sealable bags should each contain 1 1/2 cups of frozen fruit. To each bag, add 1 cup of spinach. For up to three months, freeze the sealed packets.

• Fill a blender with 1 cup milk (or a nondairy substitute) to make a smoothie. Blend the ingredients from 1 smoothie pack after adding them.

Equipment

4 freezer-safe, sealable bags, similar to Stasher Bags

Nutritional data:

One smoothie counts as one serving.

229 calories, 2g of fat, 12mg of cholesterol, 151mg of sodium, 43g of carbs, 6g of dietary fiber, 11g of

protein, 35g of sugars, 2g of saturated fat, 4793IU of vitamin A, and 366mg of potassium.

Spinach, tomato, and feta waffle

This simple and wholesome breakfast meal combines a Greek omelet with waffles. In a pinch, frozen whole-grain waffles are a fantastic breakfast option. Including nutrient-dense veggies and filling cheese will prevent hunger throughout the morning.

Flagel with goat cheese and smoked salmon

The taste of goat cheese is more robust than cream cheese. We like it spread over a Flagel (also known as a flat bagel) as a nutritious option for breakfast, brunch, or lunch.

Kefir and Raspberry Power Smoothie

Your freezer should always include ripe, peeled bananas so that you are never far from a nutritious smoothie. Protein, probiotics, and good fats are added via kefir, peanut butter, and flax meal.

Ingredients:

- 12 frozen bananas,

- 12 cups fresh or frozen raspberries,

- 13 cups plain low-fat kefir,

- 2 teaspoons natural peanut butter,

- 12 teaspoon flax meal,

- and 1 to 2 tablespoons water.

Directions

- In a blender, combine the banana, raspberries, kefir, peanut butter, and flaxseed.

- If necessary, add a tablespoon of water at a time as you process to make it smooth.

Nutritional data:

Serving Size: 1 cup Each serving contains 249 calories, 8g of protein, 40.7g of carbohydrates, 8.1g of dietary fiber, 21.5g of sugars, 7.2g of fat, 1.5g of saturated fat, 4.5mg of cholesterol, 604.1IU of vitamin A, 26.6mcg of vitamin C, 48.1mcg of folate, 137.4mg of calcium, 0.9mg of iron, 57.4mg of magnesium, 661.8mg of

Smoothie with pineapple and spinach

To counteract the bitterness of greens, use juice rather than additional sugars like honey or maple syrup. Suddenly, a serving of veggies tastes like dessert. Of course, you may use any juice that doesn't have any added sugar, like apple or orange. But this is our favorite because of the soothing pineapple taste and the ready-to-go practicality of the compact, shelf-stable cans.

Ingredients:

2 cups baby spinach, 1/4 cup pineapple juice, 1/4 cup water, 1/2 cup frozen mango chunks, and 1/2 cup frozen pineapple chunks

Direction:

Blend pineapple juice, water, spinach, mango, and pineapple in the blender. until very smooth, puree.

Nutritional data:

Serving size of one and a third cups

151 calories, 91 mg of sodium, 35g of carbs, 5g of dietary fiber, 4g of protein, 25g of sugars, and 8277IU of vitamin A.

Peanut Butter Overnight Oats with Protein

A convenient cupboard staple, the powdered peanut butter adds a wonderful vegan protein boost to smoothies and porridge. To prepare breakfast for the whole family or to meal prep breakfasts for the week, double or quadruple this recipe.

Ingredients:

Salt, 12 medium bananas, sliced, or 1/2 cup berries, 12 cups old-fashioned rolled oats (see Tip), 1 tablespoon pure maple syrup, 1 tablespoon chia seeds, 1 tablespoon powdered peanut butter, and 12 cups other plant-based milk.

In a 2-cup Mason jar, combine the soymilk (or other milk), salt, oats, syrup, chia, and powdered peanut butter. Overnight refrigerate.

• Second Step: Serve with berries or banana on top.

Nutritional data: 1 1/2 cups per serving are the serving size.

368 calories, 13.4g protein, 62.8g carbs, 10.1g dietary fiber, 21.3g sugars, 9.2g fat, 1.2g saturated fat, 318.7IU vitamin A, 5.3mg vitamin C, 48.6mcg folate, 264.1mg calcium, 3mg iron, 114.8mg magnesium, 239.5mg sodium, 0.3mg thiamin, and 12g added sugar.

Exchanges: 1 fruit, 1 lean protein, 1 other carbohydrate, 2 starches, and 12 a fat

Goat cheese and Beets Toast

This nutritious toast with beets and goat cheese is made better with a dash of lemon zest.

Banana, nut butter, and chocolate chips on a waffle

When you're pressed for time, you can quickly prepare a decadent-tasting and nutritious breakfast or snack by topping a whole-grain frozen waffle with nut butter, banana slices, and chocolate chips. You may be able to eat this high-protein, high-fiber meal before your coffee brewing.

Spinach and Kale Smoothie

When you need to consume more greens, use this smoothie, which has both kale and spinach in every serving. Dates and kiwi provide natural sweetness, while almond milk and butter help you feel full.

Nutritional Profile: Vegetarian, Vegan, Dairy-Free, Egg-Free, Gluten-Free, Soy-Free, and Healthy Pregnancy

Ingredient:

1 cup each of baby kale and spinach, 5 dates that have been pitted and coarsely chopped, 1 kiwi that has been peeled and sliced, 2 teaspoons each of creamy almond butter, and 1 cup of unsweetened vanilla almond milk

Directions:

- Fill a blender with the kale, spinach, dates, kiwi, almond butter, and almond milk. Blend until well blended at medium-low speed, using the tamper if required.
- Increase the blender's speed to medium-high and mix until extremely smooth.

Nutritional data:

419 calories, 21g of fat, 310mg of sodium, 51g of carbs, 10g of dietary fiber, 12g of protein, 36g of sugars, 2mg

of niacin equivalents, 2g of saturated fat, 5698IU of vitamin A, and 979mg of potassium.

Toast with smoked salmon and everything

For a quick and easy nutritious breakfast, spread cream cheese, smoked salmon, and everything bagel spice over your favorite whole-grain bread.

Blueberry Chia Pudding with Almonds

With this very simple chia pudding recipe, change up your typical morning porridge routine. Just like overnight oats, you mix chia with your preferred milk, let it soak overnight, then top it with sweet blueberries and salty almonds.

Nutritional Profile:

Low Sodium, High Calcium, Soy-Free, Bone Health, Healthy Aging, Healthy Pregnancy, Low Sodium, High

Fiber, Dairy-Free, Diabetes Appropriate, Egg-Free, Gluten-Free, Vegetarian, Vegan

Ingredients:

• 1 tablespoon toasted slivered almonds, divided;

• 2 tablespoons chia seeds;

• 2 teaspoons pure maple syrup;

• 18 teaspoon almond extract;

• 12 cups fresh blueberries;

• 12 cups unsweetened almond milk or other nondairy milk beverage.

Directions

• Combine the chia, maple syrup, almond extract, and almond milk (or other nondairy milk beverage) in a small bowl. For at least eight hours and up to three days, cover and chill.

• Thoroughly stir the pudding when it is time to serve. The pudding should be poured into a serving glass (or bowl) approximately halfway, and the blueberries and almonds should be placed on top. Top with the remaining blueberries and almonds and the leftover pudding mixture.

Nutritional data:

1 cup is the recommended serving size.

229 calories, 5.7g of protein, 30.3g of carbohydrates, 10.2g of dietary fiber, 15.8g of sugar, 10.8g of fat, 0.9g of saturated fat, 301.4IU of vitamin A, 7.5mcg of vitamin C, 17.3mcg of folate, 391.1mg of calcium, 2.2mg of iron, 93.2mg of magnesium, 231.1mg of potassium, 90.8mg of sodium, and 8g of added sugar.

Exchanges: two fat, one fruit, and one-half another carbohydrate

Berry-Beet Yogurt, Sweet

By combining beets and raspberry jam with plain yogurt, you can quickly and easily make a delicious and nutritious breakfast that is exploding with color. Almonds give crunch, protein, and good fats.

Toasted Greek salmon

Greek salmon toast comes with fresh dill weed and red onion that has been finely diced.

Fruit and banana smoothie with cauliflower

Every morning, have a smoothie to get your vegetables. A lightly sweetened cauliflower smoothie with the delicious notes of bananas and berries in the forefront is thickened and made creamier by the addition of riced cauliflower.

Ingredients:

• 2 cups unsweetened plain almond milk

• 1 cup frozen sliced banana

• 1/2 cup frozen mixed berries

• 1 cup frozen riced cauliflower

• 2 tablespoons maple syrup

Directions:

Blend the cauliflower, berries, banana, almond milk, and maple syrup for three to four minutes, or until the mixture is smooth.

Nutritional data: 2 cups per serving are the serving size.

149 calories, 3g of protein, 29.3g of carbohydrates, 5g of dietary fiber, 17.5g of sugar, 3g of fat, 0.1g of saturated fat, 565.8IU of vitamin A, 28.5mcg of vitamin C, 17.7mcg of folate, 473.6mg of calcium, 0.8mg of iron, 23.6mg of magnesium, 338.6mg of potassium, 184.4mg of sodium, and 4g of added sugar.

Exchanges: 1 1/2 fats, 1/2 fats, 1/2 other carbs, and 1/2 vegetables

Smoothie with bananas, peanut butter, and spinach

The traditional pairing of peanut butter and banana is made tastier by the addition of tart, probiotic-rich kefir. Additionally, the addition of a little mild-flavored spinach to this peanut butter banana smoothie helps you increase your daily vegetable servings.

Ingredients

One cup of plain kefir, one tablespoon of peanut butter, one cup of spinach, one frozen banana, and one tablespoon of honey (Optional)

Directions

In a blender, combine the kefir, peanut butter, spinach, banana, and honey (if using). Until smooth, blend.

Nutritional data:

1 1/2 cups per serving are the serving size.

324 calories, 16.3g of protein, 44.5g of carbohydrates, 5.2g of dietary fiber, 28.1g of sugars, 11.1g of fat, 3.4g of saturated fat, 13.4mg of cholesterol, 5267IU of vitamin A, 72.4mcg of folate, 415.5mg of calcium, 2.5mg of iron, 130.9mg of magnesium, 951.2mg of potassium, 219.9mg of sodium, and 1g of added sugar.

Lunch Recipe

High blood pressure is caused by an unhealthful increase in the blood flow via the blood vessels. One out of every five adults, according to the World Health Organization, has excessive blood pressure. Around 9.4 million individuals worldwide have died as a result of this common disease. Compared to countries with high incomes, this syndrome is more common in low-income nations. Hypertension may arise from a variety of causes, including genetics, environment, underlying medical conditions, hormone imbalances, and physical inactivity. The typical signs and symptoms include headaches, shortness of breath, and chest discomfort.

One has to have a healthy lifestyle in addition to eating balanced food to manage hypertension. Vegetables, fruits, lean meats, and whole grains are part of a diet that is favorable to hypertension. Here are some suggestions for healthy lunch recipes.

Dishes for lunch to lower blood pressure

Salad of broccoli: Broccoli is a well-known superfood. By encouraging the relaxation of the blood vessels, broccoli may assist those with high blood pressure decrease it. The following items are needed for this recipe:

1. Broccoli (8 cups)

• 1/4 cup sunflower seeds

• Sugar (2 tbsp)

• Rice vinegar seasoned (3 tbsp)

• Coconut oil (3 tbsp)

• Half a cup of green onions, thinly sliced

• 1/2 cup of dried cranberries

The entire preparation time for this meal, which serves 10 people, is 25 minutes. This recipe's preparation process is as follows:

• Combine the broccoli, green onions, and cranberries in a bowl.

• Use a different bowl to combine sugar, oil, and vinegar.

• Combine the components in the two bowls.

• Top the salad with sunflower seeds.

• Serve.

Chicken and quinoa make up this protein-rich meal known as the "quinoa chicken bowl." This lunch meal has great potential and might assist you in controlling your triglyceride and blood pressure levels. The following items are needed for this recipe:

• Trimmed, skinless, and boneless chicken (1 pound)

• 1/4 teaspoon of ground pepper

Oil of olives (4 tbsp)

• Red roasted peppers (1 7-ounce jar)

• 1 smashed clove of garlic

• Almonds (quarter-cup)

Salt (1/4 teaspoon)

Feta cheese (quarter cup)

• Chile (1 tsp)

• Cut up cucumber (1 cup)

• Parsley, chopped finely (2 tbsp)

• Prepared quinoa (2 cups)

• 1/4 cup of finely chopped red onions

• Ground cumin (half a teaspoon)

• Kalamata olives, pitted and chopped (2 cups)

The entire preparation time for this meal, which serves 4 people, is 30 minutes. This recipe's preparation process is as follows:

• Set a baking sheet's edge with foil and turn the broiler on high.

Salt the chicken before placing it on the baking pan.

• Broil the chicken for a minimum of 14 and a maximum of 18 minutes. Slice the chicken after bringing it to the cutting board.

• In a food processor, blend peppers, garlic, cumin, almonds, paprika, and two tablespoons of oil into a smooth puree.

• Combine quinoa, red onion, olives, and two tablespoons of oil in a bowl.

• Arrange the chicken, red pepper sauce, cucumber, and quinoa mixture on a platter in separate portions.

Serve it with feta cheese and parsley on top.

Salmon lentil salad: Salads are simple to make and provide excellent lunch menu options. Salmon, which is a high source of omega-3 fatty acids, is included in this dish. Blood pressure may be lowered by doing this. The following items are needed for this recipe:

Salt (1/4 teaspoon)

• Mustard from Dijon (2 tsp)

• Cut up cucumber (1 cup)

Lemon juice (one-third cup)

Olive oil (one-third cup)

• Dill, chopped (1/3 cup)

• Powdered pepper

• 1 red bell pepper, chopped and seeded

• 1/2 cup of red onion, finely chopped

• Cooked brown lentils (3 cups)

• 1 1/2 cups of flakes of cooked salmon

The entire preparation time for this meal, which serves 6 people, is 30 minutes. This recipe's preparation process is as follows:

• Combine the mustard, dill, pepper, salt, and lemon juice in a large bowl.

• Re-whisk after adding oil.

• Combine the bell pepper, lentils, salmon, cucumber, and onions in the bowl.

• Serve.

Dinner Recipe

A balanced high-blood pressure diet might be simpler (and tastier) to follow than you would imagine. To decrease blood pressure, we've compiled some of our tastiest dishes that can be prepared in under 25 minutes. Favorites like our Sheet-Pan Chili-Lime Salmon with Potatoes dish and the Charred Shrimp, Pesto & Quinoa Bowls are guaranteed to satisfy everyone at your table since they are rich in potassium and lower in sodium, a combination that has been proven to help support healthy blood pressure. In addition, they include a lot of herbs and spices, so even if they have less sodium, they still have a taste!

Chili-lime salmon on a sheet pan with potatoes and peppers

Simple weeknight meals, like this salmon sheet pan supper, are ideal. As the name implies, everything is prepared in a single pan. The salmon fillets with a chili coating come last after the potatoes and sweet bell peppers. It is a full dinner with little cleanup!

Ingredients

- Cut one pound of Yukon Gold potatoes into 3/4-inch chunks.
- Divide two tablespoons of extra-virgin olive oil.
- Add a three-quarters teaspoon of salt.
- Add one-fourth teaspoon of ground pepper.
- Add two teaspoons of chile powder.

Add one teaspoon of ground cumin.

- Add one-half teaspoon of garlic powder.
- 2 medium bell peppers, any color, sliced;
- 1 lime, zested and quartered
- Four halves of a center-cut,
- 1 1/4-pound salmon fillet that has been peeled, if preferred.

Directions

- Set oven to 425 degrees Fahrenheit. Spray cooking oil on a large baking sheet with a rim.

- Combine potatoes in a medium bowl with 1 tablespoon oil, 1/4 teaspoon salt, and 1/4 teaspoon pepper. After transferring, roast for 15 minutes in the preheated pan.

- In the meanwhile, mix the remaining 1/2 teaspoon salt, chili powder, cumin, garlic powder, and lime zest in a small dish. Add the remaining 1 tablespoon oil, along with 1/2 tablespoon of the spice combination, to the medium bowl of bell peppers, and toss to coat. Apply the remaining spice mixture to the fish.

- Take the pan out of the oven after 15 minutes. Stir in the peppers after adding them. 5 minutes for roasting. Remove the skillet from the oven, add part of the veggies, and then add the salmon. Roast the salmon for 6 to 8 minutes, or until it's just cooked through. slices of lime are optional.

Nutritional data

1 1/4 cups of veggies and 1 piece of fish per serving, serving size:

405 calories; 35.4g protein; 25.9g carbs; 3g dietary fiber; sugars; 17.4g fat; 2.6g saturated fat; 2.6g cholesterol; 89.6mg vitamin A; 81.4mcg folate; 45.7mg calcium; 3mg iron; 83.6mg magnesium; 1426.8mg potassium; and 516.6mg sodium.

Quinoa with Chickpea Grain Bowl

There are seeming as many different styles of grain bowls as there are stars in the sky, and there is no incorrect way to make one! However, we like to keep things traditional and straightforward with hummus, quinoa, avocado, and plenty of vegetables.

Ingredients

1 cup cooked quinoa; 1/3 cup rinsed and drained canned chickpeas; 1/2 cup cucumber slices; 1/2 cup cherry tomatoes; 1/4 avocado; 3 tablespoons hummus; 1 tablespoon finely chopped roasted red pepper; 1 tablespoon lemon juice; 1 tablespoon water; 1 teaspoon

chopped fresh parsley (optional); pinch of salt; pinch of ground pepper; and optionally, 1 teaspoon.

Directions

- Put quinoa, chickpeas, tomatoes, cucumbers, and avocado in a large bowl.
- In a bowl, combine the hummus, roasted red pepper, lemon juice, and water. To get the appropriate dressing consistency, add additional water. Stir in the parsley, salt, and pepper after adding them. With the Buddha bowl, serve.

Nutritional data

503 calories, 17.9g of protein, 75g of carbs, 16.1g of dietary fiber, 5.8g of sugar, 16.6g of fat, 2.3g of saturated fat, 1731.2IU of vitamin A, 39.3mcg of folate, 100.2mg of calcium, 5.7mg of iron, 206.1mg of magnesium, 1082mg of potassium, 1082.7mg of sodium, and 0.4mg of thiamin.

Exchanges: 1/2 carbohydrate, 1/2 medium-fat protein, 1 fat, 1 vegetable, and 4 starches.

Black bean and roasted vegetable tacos

For hectic weeknights, these meaty vegan tacos are fast and simple to prepare. No one will miss the meat or dairy since they are so delicious.

Direction

In a saucepan, mix the beans, cumin, chili powder, coriander, salt, and pepper with the roasted root vegetables. For 6 to 8 minutes, cook under cover at medium-low heat until well cooked.

Divide the mixture among the tortillas in step 2. Add avocado on top. slices of lime are optional. If desired, garnish with cilantro and/or salsa.

Nutritional data

2 tacos per serving, average serving size:

343 calories; 7.9g of protein; 44.4g of carbs; 12.1g of dietary fiber; 5.7g of sugars; 16.8g of fat; 2.4g of saturated fat; 3364.9IU of vitamin A; 12.9mcg of folate; 97.3mg of calcium; 2.7mg of iron; 64mg of magnesium; 700.8mg of potassium; and 352.4mg of sodium.

Exchanges: 1 starch, 2 1/2 fat, and 1/2 vegetable

Mixed Greens with Sliced Apple & Lentils

This lentil, feta, and apple salad is a filling vegetarian main dish that you can quickly prepare for lunch. Change to drained canned lentils to save time, but make sure to opt for low-sodium varieties and give them a rinse before incorporating them into the salad.

Ingredients

- 1 apple, cored and sliced, divided;
- 1 12 tablespoons crumbled feta cheese;
- 1 tablespoon red-wine vinegar;
- 2 teaspoons extra-virgin olive oil;

- 1 12 cups mixed salad greens;

- 12 cup cooked lentils;

Ingredients

Add lentils, roughly half the apple pieces, and feta to the greens as a garnish. Add vinegar and oil drizzle. The remaining apple slices should be served separately.

Nutritional data

3 1/2 cups per serving are the serving size.

347 calories, 12.7g of protein, 48.1g of carbohydrates, 14g of dietary fiber, 21.8g of sugar, 13.2g of fat, 3.5g of saturated fat, 12.5mg of cholesterol, 2408.7IU of vitamin A, 23.2mcg of vitamin C, 284.5mcg of folate, 145.2mg of calcium, 4.8mg of iron, 67.8mg of magnesium, 835.9mg of potassium, 154.9mg of sodium

Exchanges: 1 carbohydrate, 1/2 high-fat protein, 1/2 fruit, 1 lean protein, 2 fat, 1 1/2 fruit, 1 1/2 vegetables.

Herbed fish with mushrooms and wilted greens

This delectable and simple fish dish is perfect for a weekday supper. Serve with roasted potatoes or wild rice.

Ingredients

• 1 medium tomato, diced;

4 cups chopped kale;

• 3 tablespoons olive oil, divided;

• 12 large sweet onion, sliced;

• 3 cups sliced cremini mushrooms;

• 2 cloves garlic, sliced;

• 2 teaspoons Mediterranean Herb Mix, divided;

• 1 tablespoon lemon juice;

• 12 teaspoons salt;

• 12 teaspoon ground pepper;

Four fillets of fish, sole, or tilapia, each weighing four ounces. Fresh parsley, chopped.

Directions

- In a big saucepan, heat 1 tablespoon of oil to medium-high heat. Add the onion and simmer for 3 to 4 minutes, stirring periodically, until transparent.
- Add the mushrooms and the garlic; simmer, stirring occasionally, for 4 to 6 minutes, or until the mushrooms release their liquid and start to brown.
- Add kale, tomato, and 1 teaspoon of the herb mixture. Cook for 5 to 7 minutes, stirring periodically, or until the mushrooms are soft.
- Add lemon juice and a quarter teaspoon of each salt and pepper. Warm up, cover, and remove from heat.
- Add the remaining 1 tsp. of the herb mixture, 1/4 tsp. of salt, and 1/4 tsp. of pepper to the fish. In a big nonstick skillet over medium-high heat, warm the last 2 Tbsp of oil. Depending on

thickness, fry the fish for 2 to 4 minutes on each side or until the flesh is opaque. Placing the fish on a serving tray or four plates. Vegetables are placed on top of and around the fish; optionally, parsley is added.

Sweet potato stuffed with hummus dressing

This filled sweet potato with black beans, spinach, and hummus dressing is a filling and simple 5-ingredient lunch for one.

Directions

- Step 1: Use a fork to prick the sweet potato all over. Cook on High for 7–10 minutes, or until thoroughly heated through.
- Wash the kale in the meanwhile, allowing water to cling to the leaves as you drain it. Place in a

medium saucepan, cover, and cook until wilted while turning just occasionally over medium-high heat. If the pot is dry, add a tablespoon or two of water before adding the beans. Cook the mixture for 1 to 2 minutes with the lid off, stirring regularly, until it is boiling.

- Cut open the sweet potato, then pile the kale and bean mixture on top. In a small bowl, combine the hummus and two tablespoons of water. If more water is required to get the desired consistency, do so. Sprinkle the filled sweet potato with the hummus dressing.

Nutritional data

472 calories, 21.1g of protein, 85.3g of carbs, 22.1g of dietary fiber, 19.9g of sugar, 7g of fat, 1.2g of saturated fat, 35809.9IU of vitamin A, 55.1mcg of folate, 191mg of calcium, 6.7mg of iron, 98.9mg of magnesium, 1672.7mg of potassium, and 0.6mg of thiamin.

Exchanges: 1 medium-fat protein, 1/2 carbohydrate, 1 1/2 lean protein, and 4 starches.

Bowls of charred shrimp, pesto, and quinoa

It takes less than 30 minutes to prepare these shrimp, pesto, and quinoa bowls, which are also tasty, healthy, and attractive. They are essentially the ideal quick evening supper, to put it another way. You are welcome to add more veggies and substitute chicken, beef, tofu, or edamame for the shrimp.

Ingredient:

1 pound peeled and deveined large shrimp (16-20 count), patted dry; 4 cups arugula; 2 cups cooked quinoa; 1 cup halved cherry tomatoes; 1 avocado, diced. Ingredients: 13 cups prepared pesto; 2 tablespoons balsamic vinegar; 1 tablespoon extra-virgin olive oil; 12 teaspoon salt; 14 teaspoon ground pepper.

Directions:

- In a large bowl, stir together the pesto, vinegar, oil, salt, and pepper. To each bowl, take 4 tablespoons of the mixture, and put them both aside.
- Turn up the heat to medium-high in a large cast-iron pan. Add the shrimp and stir-fry for 4 to 5 minutes, or until just cooked through with a little char. Take out onto a platter.
- Toss the arugula and quinoa with the vinaigrette in a large bowl. The arugula mixture should be divided into 4 dishes. Add tomatoes, avocado, and shrimp on top. 1 tablespoon of the leftover pesto mixture should be drizzled over each bowl.

Nutritional data

2 1/2 cups per serving are the serving size.

429 calories, 30.9g of protein, 29.3g of carbohydrates, 7.2g of dietary fiber, 5g of sugar, 22g of fat, 3.6g of saturated fat, 187.5mg of cholesterol, 1125.6IU of vitamin A, 14.4mcg of vitamin C, 108.9mcg of folate, 205.4mg of calcium, 2.9mg of iron, 130.5mg of

magnesium, 901.1mg of potassium, 571.4mg of sodium,

Exchanges: 1 1/2 starches, 1 1/2 vegetables, 3 lean proteins, and 4 fat

Hummus and Veggie Sandwich

The ideal vegetarian meal on the go is this mile-high sandwich with hummus and vegetables. Depending on your mood, mix it up with various hummus varieties and veggies of all kinds.

Veggie & Hummus Sandwich Recipe

A sandwich with hummus and vegetables is a terrific fiber-rich option for a packed lunch. Here is our normal sandwich with a few tweaks to make it more interesting.

1.   The Bread

For our vegetable and hummus sandwich, we like the whole-grain bread's nutty taste and fiber-boosting advantages. Sandwich bread has a milder texture, so we recommend country bread or bread with a hard crust, but either can work.

2.   The Spreads

We spread our sandwich with both mashed avocado and hummus. They aid in maintaining the position of the vegetables and provide a barrier between the bread and the vegetables to help keep the bread from becoming soggy. You may add more hummus or try whipped cream cheese, either on its own or in a pesto mixture with basil or sundried tomatoes, if you don't have avocado. Just be sure to distribute it evenly over both pieces of bread. Use plain hummus or experiment with a flavor you like.

3.   The Veggies

Salad greens, shredded carrot, cucumber, and red bell pepper are just a few of the ingredients we use to make our sandwich simple. Consider adding spinach, sprouts, tomato, red onion, broccoli slaw, thinly sliced radish, and fresh herbs that are still delicate, such as basil or cilantro. However, bear in mind that briny foods like pickles and banana peppers can also add salt. Instead of stuffing the whole produce section, try to keep your variations basic and choose 3–4 vegetables. Before adding them to the sandwich, wet components like sliced tomatoes should be patted dry to eliminate more moisture.

Can I Make A Sandwich with Veggies and Hummus Ahead?

Yes! Any variant of this sandwich would be a great option for a packed lunch. The sandwich may be assembled ahead of time, chilled for up to four hours, or packed in a carry-on cooler pack with an airtight container.

Ingredients

Two pieces of whole-grain bread, three tablespoons of hummus, one-fourth of an avocado, mashed, one-half cup of mixed salad greens, one-fourth cup of sliced cucumber, and one-fourth cup of grated carrot.

Direction:

- Spread hummus on one piece of bread and avocado on the other.

- Add greens, bell pepper, cucumber, and carrot to the sandwich.

- Cut in half, then present.

Nutritional data

One sandwich per serving, serving size:

325 calories, 12.8g of protein, 39.7g of carbs, 12.1g of dietary fiber, 6.8g of sugar, 14.3g of fat, 2.2g of saturated fat, 6388.1IU of vitamin A, 49.8mcg of vitamin C, 171.1mcg of folate, 107.8mg of calcium, 3.4mg of iron, 105.3mg of magnesium, 746.3mg of potassium, 407mg of sodium, 0.3mg

Exchanges: 1 vegetable, 1/2 lean protein, 1/2 carbohydrate, 2 fat, and 1 1/2 starch.